The Mindfulness Blueprint: Techniques for Enhancing Awareness and Reducing Stress

Introduction to Mindfulness

In today's fast-paced world, many of us find ourselves overwhelmed by the constant barrage of demands and distractions. Amidst the chaos, mindfulness offers a sanctuary—a practice rooted in ancient traditions but profoundly relevant in our modern lives. At its core, mindfulness is the art of paying full attention to the present moment with openness and acceptance. It is about being aware of your thoughts, feelings, and surroundings without judgment, allowing you to experience life with greater clarity and balance.

Definition and Benefits of Mindfulness

Mindfulness can be defined as the practice of maintaining a moment-by-moment awareness of our thoughts, feelings, bodily sensations, and surrounding environment. It involves observing these aspects without reacting or getting caught up in them. Research has shown that mindfulness offers numerous benefits, including:

- Reduced Stress: By focusing on the present moment, mindfulness helps break the cycle of stress and anxiety, providing a sense of calm and relaxation.
- Improved Emotional Regulation: Mindfulness enhances your ability to manage and respond to your emotions in a balanced way, leading to increased emotional resilience.
- Enhanced Focus and Concentration: Regular mindfulness practice can sharpen your attention and improve your ability to stay focused on tasks.
- Greater Self-Awareness: Mindfulness fosters a deeper understanding of yourself, helping you recognize patterns in your thoughts and behaviors that may affect your well-being.

Overview of How Mindfulness Can Enhance Well-Being

Integrating mindfulness into your daily routine can lead to profound improvements in various aspects of your life. It encourages a more intentional and conscious way of living, where you are more in tune with your needs and experiences. Mindfulness helps you cultivate a sense of presence and appreciation, transforming ordinary moments into meaningful experiences. It also supports mental and physical health by reducing stress and promoting relaxation.

Brief Introduction to the Techniques Covered in the Book

In this book, we will explore ten practical mindfulness techniques designed to help you enhance your awareness and reduce stress. These techniques include:

1. Breathing Exercises – Simple yet powerful methods to calm the mind and body through conscious breathing.
2. Body Scan Meditation – A practice to increase bodily awareness and release tension.
3. Mindful Walking – Integrating mindfulness into the act of walking to foster presence and connection with your surroundings.
4. Loving-Kindness Meditation – Cultivating compassion and positive feelings towards yourself and others.
5. Mindful Eating – Enhancing the eating experience by focusing on the sensory aspects of food.
6. Five Senses Exercise – Grounding yourself in the present moment through sensory awareness.
7. Progressive Muscle Relaxation – Reducing physical tension through the tensing and relaxing of muscle groups.
8. Guided Imagery – Using visualization techniques to create a calming mental environment.

9. Mindful Journaling – Exploring and understanding your thoughts and feelings through writing.
10. Yoga and Tai Chi – Engaging in mindful movement practices to promote relaxation and body awareness.

Each chapter will provide detailed instructions, practical tips, and insights into how these techniques can be incorporated into your daily life. By exploring and practicing these methods, you will be equipped to cultivate a deeper sense of mindfulness and well-being.

Chapter 1: Breathing Exercises

The Power of Breath

Breathing is something we do automatically, but its impact on our physical and mental well-being is profound. When we engage in deep, mindful breathing, we stimulate the parasympathetic nervous system, which is responsible for our body's "rest and digest" functions. This activation helps counter the "fight or flight" response that stress triggers, leading to a decrease in heart rate, lower blood pressure, and a reduction in stress hormones like cortisol.

Scientific studies have shown that controlling our breath can significantly affect our stress levels and overall mental state. By focusing on our breath, we engage the autonomic nervous system, which regulates involuntary bodily functions such as heart rate and digestion. This mindful attention helps us manage stress and enter a state of calm and relaxation.

Benefits of Deep, Mindful Breathing

1. Stress Reduction: Deep breathing helps reduce stress by lowering the production of stress hormones and calming the nervous system. This promotes a sense of relaxation and tranquility.
2. Improved Focus and Concentration: Increased oxygen flow to the brain through mindful breathing enhances cognitive function and mental clarity, making it easier to focus and concentrate.
3. Enhanced Emotional Regulation: By concentrating on the breath, you create a moment of pause that allows for better management and regulation of emotions.
4. Better Physical Health: Deep breathing improves lung capacity and respiratory efficiency, contributing to overall physical health and well-being.

Techniques and Practices

Detailed Instructions on Various Breathing Exercises

1. Diaphragmatic Breathing (Belly Breathing)
   - Instructions: Find a comfortable position, either sitting or lying down. Place one hand on your chest and the other on your abdomen. Breathe deeply through your nose, allowing your abdomen to rise more than your chest. Exhale slowly through your mouth, letting your abdomen fall. Continue this for 5-10 minutes.
   - Benefits: This technique promotes relaxation by engaging the diaphragm, leading to more effective breathing and a deeper sense of calm.

2. 4-7-8 Breathing
   - Instructions: Sit or lie down in a comfortable position. Close your eyes and inhale deeply through your nose for a count of 4. Hold the breath for a count of 7. Exhale slowly through your mouth for a count of 8. Repeat this cycle for 4-6 times.
   - Benefits: This practice calms the mind and body, making it particularly useful for managing anxiety and improving sleep.

3. Box Breathing
   - Instructions: Sit or stand with your back straight. Inhale through your nose for a count of 4. Hold your breath for a count of 4. Exhale through your mouth for a count of 4. Pause and hold the breath for another count of 4 before starting the next cycle. Continue for 5-10 minutes.

- Benefits: Box breathing enhances focus and concentration, reduces stress, and stabilizes your breath rate.

4. Alternate Nostril Breathing
   - Instructions: Sit comfortably with your spine straight. Use your right thumb to close off your right nostril. Inhale deeply through your left nostril. Close the left nostril with your right ring finger and release your right nostril. Exhale through the right nostril. Inhale through the right nostril, then close it and exhale through the left nostril. Repeat this process for 5-10 minutes.
   - Benefits: This technique balances the nervous system, promotes mental clarity, and helps in reducing stress.

Tips for Integrating Breathing Practices into Daily Life

1. Set Aside Time: Designate specific times each day for your breathing exercises, such as in the morning, during breaks, or before bed. Consistent practice helps in building a routine.
2. Create Reminders: Use phone alarms or sticky notes as reminders to practice breathing exercises throughout the day, ensuring you don't forget to integrate them into your routine.
3. Combine with Other Activities: Enhance the effectiveness of your breathing exercises by integrating them with other mindfulness practices such as meditation or yoga, or use them during stressful moments.
4. Practice Mindfulness: Incorporate mindful breathing into daily activities like walking or eating. Bringing awareness to these moments can help you stay present and engaged.

Common Challenges and Solutions

Common Obstacles to Effective Breathing Practices

1. Difficulty Focusing: Many people struggle to maintain focus during breathing exercises due to a busy mind or distractions.
2. Physical Discomfort: Some may experience discomfort, such as lightheadedness or tension in the chest, while practicing deep breathing.

3. Inconsistency: Maintaining a regular practice can be challenging, especially with a busy lifestyle.

Strategies to Overcome These Challenges

1. Addressing Difficulty Focusing
   - Solution: Start with shorter sessions and gradually increase the time as you become more comfortable. Guided breathing exercises or apps can help maintain focus.
   - Solution: Create a calming environment with minimal distractions for your practice. A quiet, dedicated space can help you stay centered.

2. Managing Physical Discomfort
   - Solution: Practice breathing exercises in a comfortable position and avoid forcing the breath. If you feel lightheaded, pause and return to normal breathing.
   - Solution: Begin with gentle, shallow breaths and gradually deepen them. This approach can help your body adjust to the practice.

3. Ensuring Consistency
   - Solution: Integrate breathing exercises into your daily schedule, such as during morning or evening routines. Consistency is key to building a lasting practice.
   - Solution: Set realistic goals and track your progress to stay motivated. Joining a class or group can provide additional support and accountability.

By understanding and implementing these breathing techniques, you can harness the power of your breath to enhance your overall well-being, manage stress more effectively, and cultivate a greater sense of calm and relaxation.

Chapter 2: Body Scan Meditation

1. Understanding Body Awareness

The Importance of Connecting with Your Body

In our busy lives, we often overlook the signals our bodies send us. Body awareness involves tuning into these signals and recognizing areas of tension or discomfort. By connecting with your body, you become more attuned to its needs, which can enhance your overall well-being. Body awareness helps you understand the physical manifestations of stress, emotions, and physical strain, allowing you to address them more effectively.

How Body Scan Meditation Promotes Relaxation

Body scan meditation is a practice that involves systematically focusing on different parts of the body, bringing attention to sensations and tension. This practice promotes relaxation by:

1. Encouraging Mindfulness: It helps you stay present and aware of your bodily sensations, reducing the tendency to be distracted by thoughts or external stimuli.
2. Releasing Tension: By identifying and consciously relaxing areas of tension, body scan meditation helps release physical stress and promotes overall relaxation.
3. Enhancing Self-Awareness: Regular practice increases your awareness of bodily sensations, improving your ability to recognize and address stress or discomfort before it escalates.

2. Step-by-Step Guide

Detailed Instructions for Performing a Body Scan Meditation

1. Find a Comfortable Position
   - Lie down on your back or sit in a comfortable chair with your feet flat on the floor and your hands resting on your lap. Ensure your posture is relaxed and supported.

2. Settle into the Practice

- Close your eyes and take a few deep breaths to center yourself. Inhale deeply through your nose, allowing your abdomen to rise, and exhale slowly through your mouth, letting go of any tension.

3. Begin the Body Scan

- Start at Your Toes: Bring your attention to your toes. Notice any sensations, such as warmth, cold, or tingling. Consciously relax your toes and move your attention to the next part of your body.
- Move Upwards: Gradually shift your focus from your toes to your feet, ankles, calves, knees, thighs, and so on. Spend a few moments on each area, observing sensations and releasing tension.
- Continue Up to the Head: Progress through your abdomen, chest, back, shoulders, arms, hands, neck, and finally your head. Pay attention to any areas of discomfort or tension, and consciously relax them as you go.

4. Complete the Practice

- Once you've scanned your entire body, take a few deep breaths and bring your awareness back to the present moment. Gently open your eyes when you're ready.

5. Reflect and Conclude

- Notice how your body feels after the practice. Spend a few moments reflecting on the experience and how your body has responded.

Variations and Adaptations for Different Needs

1. Shortened Body Scan

- If you're short on time, focus on major areas of the body (e.g., feet, legs, abdomen, chest, and head) rather than every detail.

2. Focused Body Scan

- For specific issues (e.g., back pain), concentrate more on the problematic area while still performing a brief scan of the entire body.

3. Guided Body Scan

- Use a guided meditation recording or app that leads you through the body scan process, providing prompts and instructions.

3. Applications and Benefits

How to Use Body Scan Meditation for Stress Relief and Improved Health

1. Stress Relief
- Regular practice of body scan meditation helps manage stress by providing a dedicated time to focus on relaxation and bodily sensations. It can be particularly effective when used during moments of high stress or anxiety.

2. Improved Sleep
- Incorporating a body scan meditation into your pre-sleep routine can promote relaxation and improve sleep quality. It helps calm the mind and release physical tension that may interfere with restful sleep.

3. Enhanced Self-Care
- Body scan meditation fosters a deeper connection with your body, enabling you to detect and address physical discomfort or strain early. This awareness supports better self-care and can lead to healthier lifestyle choices.

4. Pain Management
- For chronic pain or discomfort, body scan meditation can be a complementary tool in managing symptoms. By focusing on the body and consciously relaxing tense areas, you may experience a reduction in pain levels and increased comfort.

By incorporating body scan meditation into your routine, you can enhance your ability to relax, improve your physical and mental well-being, and cultivate a greater awareness of your body's needs.

Chapter 3: Mindful Walking

1. The Joy of Mindful Movement

Benefits of Mindful Walking for Physical and Mental Health

Mindful walking is a simple yet profound practice that combines the benefits of physical movement with the principles of mindfulness. By bringing awareness to each step and moment, mindful walking offers several health benefits:

1. Physical Health Benefits:
   - Improved Circulation: Walking promotes cardiovascular health and enhances blood flow, contributing to overall physical well-being.
   - Increased Energy: Regular walking boosts energy levels and improves stamina.
   - Enhanced Coordination and Balance: Mindful walking can improve coordination and balance through focused movement.

2. Mental Health Benefits:
   - Stress Reduction: Mindful walking helps alleviate stress by promoting relaxation and grounding you in the present moment.
   - Enhanced Focus: The practice of paying attention to each step and sensation sharpens mental focus and concentration.
   - Emotional Well-Being: Engaging in mindful walking can elevate mood and reduce symptoms of anxiety and depression.

How It Differs from Regular Walking

Unlike regular walking, where the mind may wander or focus on distractions, mindful walking involves a deliberate and conscious awareness of each step and movement. Key differences include:

- Focused Attention: In mindful walking, you pay close attention to the sensations of walking, such as the feeling of your feet touching the ground and the rhythm of your breath.
- Intentional Movement: Each step is taken with awareness, creating a meditative quality to the act of walking.
- Present-Moment Awareness: Mindful walking emphasizes staying present and fully experiencing the moment, rather than being preoccupied with thoughts or goals.

2. Mindful Walking Practices

Instructions for Practicing Mindful Walking

1. Find a Suitable Location:
   - Choose a location that is comfortable and safe for walking. It can be a park, a quiet street, or any space where you can move freely without distractions.

2. Begin with Awareness:
   - Stand still for a moment, taking a few deep breaths to center yourself. Notice your body's connection to the ground and your breathing pattern.

3. Start Walking Slowly:
   - Begin walking at a slow and deliberate pace. Pay attention to each step, feeling the ground beneath your feet and the movement of your legs.

4. Focus on Sensations:
   - Bring your attention to the sensations in your body as you walk. Notice the shift of weight, the feeling of your feet lifting and landing, and the movement of your arms.

5. Incorporate Breathing:
   - Synchronize your breath with your steps. For example, you might inhale for three steps and exhale for three steps, maintaining a steady rhythm.

6. Stay Present:

- If your mind starts to wander, gently bring your focus back to the act of walking and the sensations you are experiencing. Use your breath or the feeling of your feet touching the ground as anchors.

7. Conclude with Reflection:
   - When you finish your mindful walk, take a moment to pause and reflect on the experience. Notice how you feel physically and mentally.

Suggestions for Incorporating Mindful Walking into Your Routine

1. Daily Practice:
   - Integrate mindful walking into your daily routine, such as during your commute, lunch break, or evening stroll.

2. Walking Meetings:
   - Consider having walking meetings or discussions while practicing mindful walking, especially if you work in an environment where meetings are held.

3. Mindful Breaks:
   - Use mindful walking as a break during your workday or study sessions to refresh your mind and reduce stress.

4. Combine with Other Practices:
   - Pair mindful walking with other mindfulness practices, such as mindful breathing or body scan meditation, to deepen your overall mindfulness experience.

3. Real-Life Applications

Using Mindful Walking in Various Settings

1. Parks and Nature Trails:

- Parks and natural settings are ideal for mindful walking, providing a serene environment that enhances the practice. Pay attention to the natural surroundings, such as the sound of birds or the rustle of leaves.

2. Urban Environments:
   - Mindful walking can be practiced in urban settings, such as streets or plazas. Focus on the sensations of walking and the urban environment, and observe the rhythm of city life without getting caught up in it.

3. Indoor Spaces:
   - If outdoor walking is not possible, practice mindful walking indoors, such as in a large room or hallway. Use this opportunity to connect with your body and breath in a contained space.

4. During Travel:
   - Use mindful walking as a way to stay grounded and reduce stress during travel. Whether in an airport, train station, or hotel, take moments to walk mindfully and stay present.

By incorporating mindful walking into your daily routine and various settings, you can cultivate a deeper connection with your body and the present moment, enhancing both physical and mental well-being.

Chapter 4: Loving-Kindness Meditation

1. Cultivating Compassion

The Psychological and Emotional Benefits of Loving-Kindness

Loving-kindness meditation, also known as "metta" meditation, is a practice designed to cultivate compassion and unconditional love towards oneself and others. This meditation technique has profound psychological and emotional benefits, including:

1. Enhanced Emotional Well-Being:
   - Loving-kindness meditation fosters positive emotions such as love, empathy, and joy. Practicing regularly can help reduce negative emotions like anger, resentment, and sadness.

2. Improved Resilience:
   - By cultivating a compassionate mindset, individuals become more resilient to life's challenges. Loving-kindness meditation strengthens emotional resilience and helps in managing stress and adversity.

3. Reduced Self-Criticism:
   - Practicing loving-kindness towards oneself helps to counteract self-critical thoughts and promotes a more positive self-image. It encourages self-acceptance and self-compassion.

4. Enhanced Relationship Quality:
   - Loving-kindness meditation improves interpersonal relationships by fostering empathy, patience, and understanding. It helps in resolving conflicts and building stronger connections with others.

How It Impacts Relationships and Self-Esteem

1. Relationships:
   - By practicing loving-kindness, you develop a greater capacity for empathy and forgiveness. This can lead to more harmonious and fulfilling relationships, as you become more attuned to the needs and feelings of others.

2. Self-Esteem:
   - Loving-kindness meditation promotes self-compassion and acceptance, which boosts self-esteem. When you approach yourself with kindness and understanding, you are more likely to develop a healthy sense of self-worth.

2. Guided Loving-Kindness Practices

Step-by-Step Instructions for Conducting Loving-Kindness Meditation

1. Find a Comfortable Position:
   - Sit comfortably in a quiet space. You can sit on a chair, cushion, or the floor, ensuring that your back is straight and your posture is relaxed.

2. Begin with Yourself:
   - Close your eyes and take a few deep breaths to center yourself. Focus on generating a feeling of warmth and kindness towards yourself. Silently repeat phrases such as, "May I be happy," "May I be healthy," "May I be safe," and "May I live with ease."

3. Expand to Others:
   - Once you have established a feeling of kindness towards yourself, gradually extend these feelings to others. Start with someone you care about, such as a friend or family member. Repeat similar phrases for them, such as, "May [Name] be happy," "May [Name] be healthy," "May [Name] be safe," and "May [Name] live with ease."

4. Include Neutral and Difficult People:
   - Extend loving-kindness to neutral individuals (e.g., acquaintances) and eventually to those with whom you may have conflicts or difficulties. Offer them the same wishes of happiness and well-being.

5. Conclude with the World:
   - Finally, extend your loving-kindness to all beings everywhere. Imagine sending love and compassion to everyone in the world, wishing them happiness and peace.

6. Reflect and Close:
   - Take a few moments to reflect on the practice and how you feel. Gently open your eyes and return to your day with a sense of warmth and compassion.

Variations for Different Levels of Experience

1. Shortened Practice:
   - For those new to meditation or with limited time, start with a brief session, focusing on just yourself and one or two loved ones.

2. Guided Meditation:
   - Use guided meditation recordings or apps that provide structured instructions and prompts for loving-kindness practice.

3. Focused Themes:
   - Incorporate specific themes or goals, such as practicing loving-kindness during challenging situations or focusing on particular relationships.

3. Integrating into Daily Life

Practical Ways to Incorporate Loving-Kindness into Interactions and Self-Reflection

1. Daily Reminders:
   - Set reminders throughout your day to pause and send yourself or others thoughts of loving-kindness. Use sticky notes, phone alarms, or simple mental cues.

2. Mindful Interactions:
   - Practice loving-kindness during interactions with others by being present, patient, and empathetic. Approach conversations with the intention of understanding and supporting the other person.

3. Self-Compassion Practices:
   - Integrate loving-kindness into your self-care routine by acknowledging and addressing self-criticism with compassionate self-talk. Practice self-kindness during moments of self-doubt or challenge.

4. Journaling:
   - Reflect on your experiences with loving-kindness in a journal. Write about how the practice affects your interactions and emotional state, and explore any insights gained.

5. Acts of Kindness:
   - Extend the practice of loving-kindness beyond meditation by engaging in acts of kindness towards others. Small gestures of kindness, such as a compliment or helping hand, can reinforce your compassionate mindset.

By incorporating loving-kindness meditation into your daily routine and interactions, you can cultivate a deeper sense of compassion, enhance your emotional well-being, and foster more meaningful connections with others.

Chapter 5: Mindful Eating

1. The Art of Eating Mindfully

Benefits of Mindful Eating for Digestion and Overall Health

Mindful eating is the practice of paying full attention to the experience of eating and drinking, both inside and outside the body. This approach offers numerous benefits for digestion and overall health:

1. Improved Digestion:
   - Eating mindfully helps you chew food thoroughly and eat slowly, which aids in better digestion and nutrient absorption. This can reduce issues such as bloating and indigestion.

2. Enhanced Satiety:
   - By eating slowly and paying attention to your body's hunger and fullness signals, you are more likely to recognize when you are satisfied, which can help prevent overeating and promote healthy weight management.

3. Better Food Choices:

- Mindful eating encourages you to be more aware of the quality and source of your food, leading to healthier food choices and a greater appreciation for the nutrients your body needs.

4. Emotional Well-Being:
   - Engaging in mindful eating can help reduce emotional eating and increase your connection to the present moment, leading to a more positive relationship with food.

How It Enhances the Eating Experience

1. Increased Awareness:
   - Mindful eating heightens your awareness of the flavors, textures, and aromas of your food, making each meal more enjoyable and satisfying.

2. Heightened Appreciation:
   - By fully experiencing and savoring each bite, you develop a greater appreciation for the food you eat, enhancing your overall eating experience.

3. Deeper Connection:
   - Mindful eating fosters a deeper connection between your body, mind, and food, promoting a holistic approach to nourishment and well-being.

2. Mindful Eating Techniques

Instructions for Mindful Eating Practices

1. Start with Gratitude:
   - Before eating, take a moment to express gratitude for your meal. Acknowledge the effort that went into preparing the food and the nourishment it provides.

2. Eat Slowly and Deliberately:
   - Take small bites and chew each bite thoroughly. Pay attention to the taste, texture, and temperature of the food as you eat.

3. Focus on the Present Moment:
   - Avoid distractions such as TV or smartphones. Instead, concentrate on the sensory experience of eating and the signals your body is sending you.

4. Savor Each Bite:
   - Notice the flavors and textures of your food. Take time to fully experience each bite and appreciate the different components of your meal.

5. Listen to Your Body:
   - Pay attention to your hunger and fullness cues. Eat until you are satisfied, not until you are full or overstuffed.

Tips for Overcoming Common Challenges

1. Eating Too Quickly:
   - Set a timer for 20 minutes and use this as a guideline for how long you should spend eating your meal. This can help you slow down and focus on your food.

2. Distractions:
   - Create a designated eating space free from distractions. Turn off screens and avoid multitasking while eating to maintain focus on your meal.

3. Emotional Eating:
   - Practice self-awareness and recognize triggers for emotional eating. Use mindful eating techniques to address emotional cravings and develop healthier eating habits.

4. Mindless Snacking:
   - Apply mindful eating principles to snacks by being intentional about what you eat and how you eat it. Choose snacks that nourish your body and consume them with full attention.

3. Creating a Mindful Eating Environment

How to Set Up Your Eating Space for Mindfulness

1. Designate a Eating Area:
   - Create a specific space for eating that is clean, organized, and free from clutter. This helps create a calm environment conducive to mindful eating.

2. Use Simple Tableware:
   - Choose tableware that enhances your eating experience without causing distraction. Simple, visually pleasing dishes can help you focus on the food.

3. Create a Calm Atmosphere:
   - Set the mood for mindful eating with soft lighting, calming music, or a pleasant aroma. This can help you relax and enjoy your meal.

Suggestions for Mindful Eating at Home and on the Go

1. At Home:
   - Plan and prepare meals mindfully by choosing fresh, wholesome ingredients. Take time to set the table and create a peaceful eating environment.

2. On the Go:
   - When eating out or eating on the go, make an effort to stay present. Take a moment to appreciate the food before you eat and avoid rushing through meals.

3. Mindful Snacking:
   - Carry healthy snacks and practice mindful eating even during snack time. Pause to appreciate the flavor and texture of your snacks and eat them with intention.

4. Meal Prep with Awareness:
   - Approach meal preparation as an opportunity for mindfulness. Be present during the cooking process and savor the anticipation of your meal.

By incorporating mindful eating practices into your daily routine, you can enhance your overall health, deepen your enjoyment of food, and cultivate a more balanced and mindful relationship with what you eat.

Chapter 6: Five Senses Exercise

1. Grounding Through the Senses

The Role of Sensory Awareness in Mindfulness

Sensory awareness is a fundamental aspect of mindfulness, as it anchors us to the present moment and helps cultivate a deeper connection with our surroundings. By focusing on our senses, we can break free from habitual thought patterns and immerse ourselves fully in our experiences. This grounding technique involves:

1. Heightened Presence:
   - Paying attention to our senses draws our focus away from past regrets or future anxieties, bringing our awareness to the here and now.

2. Enhanced Connection:
   - Engaging our senses helps us connect more deeply with our environment, fostering a greater appreciation for the nuances of our surroundings.

3. Increased Awareness:
   - Sensory awareness enhances our ability to notice subtle details and sensations, enriching our overall experience of life.

Benefits of Engaging All Five Senses

1. Reduced Stress:
   - By grounding ourselves in sensory experiences, we can alleviate stress and anxiety, providing a calming effect on the mind and body.

2. Improved Emotional Regulation:
   - Sensory awareness helps regulate emotions by focusing attention away from overwhelming thoughts and toward the immediate sensory experience.

3. Enhanced Enjoyment:
   - Fully engaging our senses can lead to a greater enjoyment of everyday activities, making ordinary moments more vivid and satisfying.

4. Mindful Living:
   - Regular practice of sensory awareness encourages a mindful approach to life, promoting a sense of presence and contentment.

2. The Five Senses Exercise

Detailed Guide for Practicing the Five Senses Exercise

1. Find a Comfortable Position:
   - Sit or stand in a comfortable position where you can relax and focus on your surroundings. You may choose to close your eyes or keep them open, depending on your preference.

2. Start with the Sense of Sight:
   - Take a moment to observe your environment. Notice five things you can see, paying attention to colors, shapes, and details.

3. Move to the Sense of Touch:
   - Focus on your sense of touch. Identify four things you can feel, such as the texture of your clothing, the surface you are sitting on, or the feeling of the air against your skin.

4. Notice the Sense of Hearing:
   - Pay attention to the sounds around you. Listen for three distinct noises, whether they are distant or nearby, and note their qualities and patterns.

5. Engage the Sense of Smell:
   - Tune into your sense of smell. Identify two different scents in your environment, such as the aroma of food, the scent of flowers, or even the smell of the air.

6. Focus on the Sense of Taste:
   - Finally, bring awareness to your sense of taste. If you are eating or drinking, notice the flavors. If not, consider the lingering taste in your mouth or simply the sensation of your tongue.

7. Reflect and Conclude:
   - Take a moment to reflect on the exercise. Notice how engaging your senses has affected your state of mind and overall awareness.

Tips for Enhancing Sensory Awareness

1. Practice Regularly:
   - Incorporate the five senses exercise into your daily routine to build and maintain heightened sensory awareness.

2. Use Mindful Reminders:
   - Set reminders throughout the day to pause and engage your senses, especially during moments of stress or distraction.

3. Create a Sensory Journal:
   - Keep a journal to record your sensory observations and experiences. Reflecting on these entries can deepen your practice and awareness.

4. Engage with Nature:
   - Spend time in natural settings where sensory experiences are rich and varied. Nature offers a wealth of sensory stimuli that can enhance mindfulness.

3. Practical Applications

How to Use This Exercise in Various Situations

1. During Stressful Moments:
   - When feeling overwhelmed or stressed, use the five senses exercise to ground yourself. Focusing on sensory experiences can help shift your attention away from stressors and into the present moment.

2. In Moments of Anxiety:
   - Practice the five senses exercise as a way to manage anxiety. Engaging your senses can provide immediate relief and help you regain a sense of calm.

3. For Relaxation:
   - Use the exercise as part of a relaxation routine. Engaging your senses mindfully can deepen your sense of relaxation and enhance your overall well-being.

4. While Eating:
   - Apply the five senses exercise to meals to enhance mindful eating. Fully engaging with the sensory aspects of your food can increase your enjoyment and promote better digestion.

5. In Daily Activities:
   - Integrate sensory awareness into routine activities such as walking, cleaning, or commuting. By practicing the five senses exercise in everyday tasks, you can cultivate a more mindful approach to daily life.

By regularly practicing the five senses exercise, you can foster greater awareness, reduce stress, and enhance your overall experience of life. This simple yet powerful technique can be a valuable tool for cultivating mindfulness and connecting more deeply with the world around you.

Chapter 7: Progressive Muscle Relaxation

1. Understanding Muscle Tension

The Connection Between Muscle Tension and Stress

Muscle tension is a common physical response to stress and anxiety. When we experience stress, our body often reacts with a "fight-or-flight" response, which includes the tightening of muscles. This tension can become chronic and contribute to physical discomfort, pain, and overall stress. Understanding this connection is crucial for managing stress effectively.

1. Physical Response to Stress:
   - When stressed, muscles contract as part of the body's natural response. Common areas of tension include the shoulders, neck, jaw, and back.

2. Chronic Muscle Tension:
   - Prolonged stress can lead to chronic muscle tension, which may result in stiffness, pain, and reduced flexibility. This can also affect posture and contribute to discomfort.

3. Impact on Well-Being:
   - Chronic muscle tension can exacerbate feelings of stress and anxiety, create a cycle of physical and emotional discomfort, and negatively impact overall well-being.

Benefits of Progressive Muscle Relaxation

Progressive Muscle Relaxation (PMR) is a technique designed to help break the cycle of muscle tension by systematically tensing and then relaxing different muscle groups. This practice offers several benefits:

1. Stress Reduction:

- PMR helps to alleviate physical and mental stress by promoting deep relaxation and reducing overall muscle tension.

2. Improved Sleep:
   - Regular practice of PMR can improve sleep quality by calming the nervous system and preparing the body for restful sleep.

3. Enhanced Body Awareness:
   - PMR increases awareness of muscle tension and relaxation, helping you recognize and address tension more effectively in daily life.

4. Pain Relief:
   - By reducing muscle tension, PMR can provide relief from tension-related pain, such as headaches and back pain.

2. Step-by-Step Guide

Detailed Instructions for Progressive Muscle Relaxation

1. Find a Comfortable Position:
   - Sit or lie down in a comfortable position where you can fully relax. Ensure your body is supported and that you are in a quiet environment.

2. Begin with Deep Breathing:
   - Start with a few deep breaths to center yourself. Inhale deeply through your nose, allowing your abdomen to rise, and exhale slowly through your mouth.

3. Tense and Relax Each Muscle Group:
   - Begin with your feet and work your way up to your head. For each muscle group, follow these steps:

- Feet: Curl your toes downward and tighten the muscles in your feet. Hold the tension for 5-10 seconds, then release and let the muscles relax completely. Notice the contrast between tension and relaxation.

- Calves: Tighten the muscles in your calves by flexing your feet upward. Hold for 5-10 seconds, then release and relax.

- Thighs: Squeeze your thighs together and tense the muscles. Hold for 5-10 seconds, then relax.

- Buttocks: Clench your buttocks muscles tightly. Hold for 5-10 seconds, then release.

- Abdomen: Tighten your abdominal muscles. Hold for 5-10 seconds, then relax.

- Chest: Take a deep breath and puff out your chest, tensing the muscles. Hold for 5-10 seconds, then release.

- Arms: Tighten your fists and flex your arms. Hold for 5-10 seconds, then relax.

- Shoulders: Shrug your shoulders up towards your ears and hold the tension. Release and let your shoulders drop.

- Neck: Gently tilt your head back and tense the muscles in your neck. Hold for 5-10 seconds, then relax.

- Face: Clench your jaw, close your eyes tightly, and frown. Hold for 5-10 seconds, then relax.

4. Complete the Practice:
- After relaxing each muscle group, take a few moments to enjoy the sensation of complete relaxation. Notice how your body feels after the practice.

Variations for Different Muscle Groups

1. Shortened Practice:
   - If time is limited, focus on key muscle groups such as shoulders, neck, and jaw. This can still provide significant relaxation benefits.

2. Targeted Tension:
   - Address specific areas of tension by dedicating extra time to those muscle groups. For example, if you have chronic back pain, spend additional time on the back muscles.

3. Mindful Integration:
   - Combine PMR with other mindfulness practices, such as deep breathing or guided imagery, to enhance the relaxation experience.

3. Incorporating into Routine

How to Integrate This Practice into Daily Life

1. Regular Practice:
   - Incorporate PMR into your daily routine, such as in the morning, before bed, or during breaks. Regular practice helps maintain muscle relaxation and stress management.

2. Pre-Sleep Routine:
   - Use PMR as part of your bedtime routine to help relax your body and mind before sleep. This can improve sleep quality and promote restful sleep.

3. Stressful Situations:
   - Practice PMR during stressful situations or when feeling tense. Even a brief session can help calm your body and mind.

4. Workplace Integration:

- Practice PMR during work breaks to alleviate stress and muscle tension. Short sessions can be done discreetly at your desk or in a quiet space.

Tips for Using Progressive Muscle Relaxation Effectively

1. Consistency:
   - Practice PMR consistently to build and maintain relaxation skills. Aim for regular sessions to reinforce the benefits.

2. Comfort and Environment:
   - Ensure that you are in a comfortable and quiet environment where you can fully relax. Create a calming atmosphere to enhance the practice.

3. Mindful Focus:
   - Stay focused on the sensations of tension and relaxation in each muscle group. Avoid distractions and maintain a mindful awareness throughout the practice.

4. Adapt as Needed:
   - Modify the practice to suit your needs and preferences. Experiment with different muscle groups and durations to find what works best for you.

By incorporating Progressive Muscle Relaxation into your routine, you can effectively manage muscle tension, reduce stress, and promote overall well-being. This practice helps you cultivate a greater sense of relaxation and physical comfort, contributing to a more balanced and mindful life.

Chapter 8: Guided Imagery

1. The Power of Visualization

Benefits of Guided Imagery for Relaxation and Mental Clarity

Guided imagery is a relaxation technique that involves using the imagination to create calming and positive mental images. This practice leverages the power of visualization to enhance relaxation, reduce stress, and improve mental clarity. The benefits of guided imagery include:

1. Deep Relaxation:
   - Guided imagery helps induce a state of deep relaxation by allowing the mind to escape from everyday stressors and immerse itself in soothing mental imagery.

2. Stress Reduction:
   - Visualization can lower stress levels by promoting relaxation and reducing the physiological effects of stress, such as increased heart rate and muscle tension.

3. Enhanced Mental Clarity:
   - By focusing the mind on positive and calming images, guided imagery can clear mental clutter, improve concentration, and foster a sense of mental clarity.

4. Improved Emotional Well-Being:
   - Engaging in positive visualization can enhance mood, increase feelings of well-being, and foster a more optimistic outlook.

How Visualization Affects the Mind and Body

1. Mental Imagery:
   - Visualization engages the brain's sensory and emotional centers, creating vivid mental images that can affect mood and physiological responses.

2. Relaxation Response:
   - Imagining calming scenes or situations can trigger the body's relaxation response, reducing the production of stress hormones and promoting a state of calm.

3. Emotional Impact:
   - Positive imagery can elicit emotional responses such as happiness and contentment, which can counteract negative emotions and improve overall emotional health.

4. Physiological Effects:
   - Visualization can influence physical processes, such as lowering blood pressure and reducing muscle tension, by promoting relaxation and altering stress responses.

2. Guided Imagery Techniques

Instructions for Practicing Guided Imagery

1. Prepare Your Space:
   - Find a quiet, comfortable place where you can relax without interruptions. Sit or lie down in a position that allows you to be at ease.

2. Begin with Relaxation:
   - Take a few deep breaths to center yourself. Inhale deeply through your nose, allowing your abdomen to rise, and exhale slowly through your mouth.

3. Select a Scene or Image:
   - Choose a calming and pleasant image or scene to focus on. This could be a peaceful beach, a serene forest, or a cozy room.

4. Create Vivid Details:
   - Close your eyes and begin to visualize the chosen scene. Engage all your senses by imagining the sights, sounds, smells, and sensations of the environment.

5. Immerse Yourself:
   - Allow yourself to fully immerse in the visualization. Imagine yourself in the scene, interacting with the environment and experiencing the sensations as if they were real.

6. Enhance the Experience:
   - Add details to make the imagery more vivid. For example, if you are visualizing a beach, imagine the warmth of the sun, the sound of waves, and the feeling of sand beneath your feet.

7. Maintain Focus:
   - If your mind wanders, gently bring your focus back to the visualization. Use deep breathing to stay centered and enhance the calming effect.

8. Conclude the Practice:
   - After spending a few minutes in your visualization, gradually bring your awareness back to the present moment. Take a few deep breaths and open your eyes.

Creating Personalized Guided Imagery Scripts

1. Identify Your Needs:
   - Determine what you want to achieve with your guided imagery practice. This could include relaxation, stress relief, or improved focus.

2. Craft a Script:
   - Write a personalized guided imagery script based on your needs. Include specific details about the scene or situation you want to visualize. For example, if you want to relax, describe a peaceful beach scene with calming sounds and sensations.

3. Use Descriptive Language:
   - Use vivid and descriptive language in your script to create a clear and engaging mental image. Focus on sensory details to make the imagery more immersive.

4. Record or Read Aloud:
   - You can record your script or read it aloud to yourself during the practice. This helps guide your visualization and ensures you stay focused on the imagery.

5. Adapt as Needed:

- Modify your script as needed to suit different situations or preferences. Experiment with various scenes and details to find what works best for you.

3. Applications in Stress Management

Using Guided Imagery for Specific Stress-Related Scenarios

1. Workplace Stress:
   - Use guided imagery to create a mental escape from workplace stress. Visualize a calming environment or a successful outcome to help manage job-related anxiety.

2. Performance Anxiety:
   - For performance-related stress, visualize yourself succeeding and feeling confident. Imagine the positive outcomes and your ability to handle challenges effectively.

3. General Stress Relief:
   - Practice guided imagery to alleviate general stress. Visualize relaxing scenarios, such as a tranquil garden or a peaceful lake, to help reduce overall stress levels.

4. Pre-Sleep Routine:
   - Use guided imagery as part of your bedtime routine to promote relaxation and prepare your mind and body for restful sleep. Visualize calming scenes or peaceful settings to ease into sleep.

Enhancing the Effectiveness of Imagery Practices

1. Consistency:
   - Practice guided imagery regularly to reinforce its benefits and improve its effectiveness over time.

2. Personalization:
   - Tailor your visualizations to your personal preferences and needs. The more relevant and engaging the imagery, the more effective it will be.

3. Combine with Other Techniques:
   - Integrate guided imagery with other relaxation techniques, such as deep breathing or progressive muscle relaxation, to enhance overall stress management.

4. Create a Ritual:
   - Establish a routine or ritual around your guided imagery practice to make it a regular and valued part of your self-care routine.

By incorporating guided imagery into your stress management practices, you can harness the power of visualization to achieve relaxation, mental clarity, and emotional well-being. This technique offers a versatile and effective approach to managing stress and enhancing overall quality of life.

Chapter 9: Mindful Journaling

1. Exploring Inner Thoughts

Benefits of Journaling for Emotional Insight and Stress Relief

Mindful journaling is a powerful tool for self-exploration, emotional insight, and stress relief. By engaging in this practice, individuals can gain a deeper understanding of their thoughts and feelings, leading to greater emotional clarity and well-being. Here are some key benefits of mindful journaling:

1. Emotional Insight:
   - Journaling allows individuals to explore and articulate their emotions, leading to a better understanding of their emotional landscape. This self-awareness can help identify patterns, triggers, and underlying issues.

2. Stress Relief:

- Writing about thoughts and feelings can serve as a form of emotional release, reducing stress and anxiety. It provides an outlet for processing and managing difficult emotions.

3. Clarity and Focus:
   - Mindful journaling helps to clarify thoughts and organize them in a coherent manner. This process can enhance focus and decision-making by providing a structured way to reflect on issues.

4. Self-Reflection and Growth:
   - Regular journaling encourages self-reflection, fostering personal growth and development. It allows individuals to track progress, set goals, and evaluate their experiences over time.

How Mindful Journaling Differs from Regular Journaling

1. Intentional Awareness:
   - Mindful journaling emphasizes present-moment awareness and intentional reflection. Unlike regular journaling, which may be more stream-of-consciousness or goal-oriented, mindful journaling focuses on being fully present with one's thoughts and feelings.

2. Deep Reflection:
   - Mindful journaling often involves exploring deeper emotional and cognitive processes. It encourages writers to delve into the underlying causes of their feelings and thoughts, rather than just noting surface-level observations.

3. Non-Judgmental Approach:
   - Mindful journaling promotes a non-judgmental attitude towards one's writing. It encourages acceptance and curiosity about one's thoughts, rather than self-criticism or evaluation.

4. Presence and Awareness:

- This practice involves a heightened awareness of the writing process itself. Writers are encouraged to focus on their sensory experiences, such as the feel of the pen or the rhythm of their writing, to enhance the mindfulness aspect.

2. Mindful Journaling Practices

Instructions for Effective Mindful Journaling

1. Create a Quiet Space:
   - Find a calm and comfortable place where you can write without distractions. This could be a dedicated journaling corner, a cozy chair, or any space where you feel at ease.

2. Set Aside Time:
   - Allocate a specific time each day or week for journaling. Consistency helps to make mindful journaling a regular and valued practice.

3. Begin with Deep Breathing:
   - Before you start writing, take a few deep breaths to center yourself. Focus on your breath and let go of any distractions or stress.

4. Write with Awareness:
   - Start writing about whatever is present in your mind and emotions. Allow yourself to explore thoughts and feelings without censorship or judgment.

5. Use Descriptive Language:
   - When journaling, use descriptive language to capture your experiences and emotions. Describe how you feel, what you are thinking, and the physical sensations you are experiencing.

6. Practice Non-Judgment:
   - Approach your writing with a non-judgmental attitude. Accept whatever comes up in your journal without self-criticism or evaluation.

7. Reflect and Review:
   - After writing, take a few moments to reflect on what you have written. Consider any insights or patterns that emerge and how they might inform your understanding of yourself.

Prompts and Exercises for Deeper Reflection

1. Emotional Check-In:
   - Write about how you are feeling in the present moment. Describe the emotions you are experiencing and any physical sensations associated with them.

2. Gratitude Reflection:
   - List three things you are grateful for today. Explore why these things are significant and how they contribute to your well-being.

3. Daily Highlights:
   - Reflect on the most meaningful or noteworthy aspects of your day. Describe what happened, how it made you feel, and any insights gained.

4. Self-Compassion Exercise:
   - Write a letter to yourself with kindness and understanding. Offer support and compassion for any challenges or difficulties you are facing.

5. Future Aspirations:
   - Explore your goals and aspirations. Write about what you want to achieve, why it is important to you, and the steps you can take to reach these goals.

3. Incorporating into Daily Life

How to Make Journaling a Regular Practice

1. Establish a Routine:

- Create a consistent journaling routine by setting aside a specific time each day or week. Whether it's in the morning, before bed, or during lunch breaks, find a time that works best for you.

2. Use a Journal You Love:

- Choose a journal that you find aesthetically pleasing and enjoyable to write in. This can make the journaling experience more inviting and engaging.

3. Set Realistic Goals:

- Start with small, manageable goals for your journaling practice. You might aim for just five minutes of writing each day or a few entries per week.

4. Make It a Ritual:

- Incorporate journaling into a larger self-care routine. For example, pair it with a cup of tea or a calming environment to enhance the practice.

Tips for Overcoming Writer's Block and Maintaining Consistency

1. Start Small:

- If you experience writer's block, start with brief entries or simple prompts. Gradually build up to longer or more complex reflections as you feel more comfortable.

2. Be Patient with Yourself:

- Allow yourself to write imperfectly. The goal is not to produce polished writing but to engage with your thoughts and emotions authentically.

3. Change Your Approach:

- If you find yourself stuck, try changing your journaling approach. Experiment with different prompts, writing styles, or journaling formats to find what works for you.

4. Keep It Accessible:

- Carry a small journal or use a digital app to jot down thoughts and reflections throughout the day. This can help you capture insights whenever they arise.

5. Celebrate Progress:
   - Acknowledge and celebrate the progress you make with your journaling practice. Reflect on any insights or growth you've experienced as a result of your writing.

By incorporating mindful journaling into your routine, you can cultivate a deeper understanding of your inner world, enhance emotional well-being, and manage stress more effectively. This practice offers a valuable tool for self-reflection and personal growth, fostering a greater connection with yourself and your experiences.

Chapter 10: Yoga and Tai Chi

1. Mindful Movement Practices

Benefits of Yoga and Tai Chi for Body Awareness and Relaxation

Yoga and tai chi are both excellent practices for enhancing body awareness and achieving relaxation. Here's how each contributes to these benefits:

1. Yoga:
   - Body Awareness: Yoga helps individuals become more attuned to their physical sensations through its diverse range of postures and stretches. Each pose requires awareness of body alignment, balance, and flexibility.
   - Relaxation: The practice of yoga incorporates deep breathing and mindful movement, which can lower stress levels and promote a sense of calm. Many yoga sessions end with a relaxation pose, such as Savasana, that helps consolidate the benefits of the practice.

2. Tai Chi:

- Body Awareness: Tai chi's slow, flowing movements improve coordination and balance, enhancing overall body awareness. The practice emphasizes the connection between mind and body, making practitioners more aware of their physical presence.
- Relaxation: Tai chi promotes relaxation through its gentle, meditative movements. The focus on breathing and smooth transitions between movements reduces stress and encourages mental tranquility.

Differences and Similarities Between Yoga and Tai Chi

1. Similarities:
  - Mindfulness: Both practices emphasize mindfulness, requiring practitioners to focus on the present moment and their bodily sensations.
  - Breath Control: Yoga and tai chi use breath control to enhance movement and relaxation. In yoga, breathing techniques often accompany specific poses, while in tai chi, breath is synchronized with fluid movements.
  - Flow and Movement: Both involve continuous, deliberate movements. Yoga's sequences involve transitioning from one pose to another, while tai chi features flowing movements that are part of a larger form or sequence.

2. Differences:
  - Origin and Philosophy:
    - Yoga: Originates from ancient India and encompasses physical postures (asanas), breath control (pranayama), and meditation. It includes a broader spiritual and philosophical context.
    - Tai Chi: Originates from ancient China and is a martial art practiced for its health benefits. It involves slow, deliberate movements and emphasizes the concept of Qi (internal energy).
  - Movement Style:
    - Yoga: Focuses on holding static postures that stretch and strengthen different parts of the body. Each pose is held for a period of time, allowing for deep stretching and strengthening.
    - Tai Chi: Involves continuous, flowing movements performed in a sequence. The practice emphasizes smooth transitions and coordination, often with a martial arts component.

2. Yoga and Tai Chi Techniques

Basic Instructions for Key Poses and Movements in Yoga and Tai Chi

Yoga Techniques:

1. Mountain Pose (Tadasana):
   - Instructions: Stand with feet together or hip-width apart. Distribute your weight evenly across both feet. Engage your thighs, lift your chest, and reach your arms overhead, with palms facing each other or touching. Hold the pose for a few breaths, focusing on grounding and alignment.
   - Benefits: Improves posture, strengthens thighs, and increases body awareness.

2. Downward-Facing Dog (Adho Mukha Svanasana):
   - Instructions: Start on hands and knees. Lift your hips towards the ceiling, straightening your legs and forming an inverted V shape. Press your heels towards the ground and extend your arms forward, spreading your fingers wide. Hold for several breaths, focusing on stretching the spine and hamstrings.
   - Benefits: Stretches the entire back, strengthens arms and legs, and improves circulation.

3. Warrior II (Virabhadrasana II):
   - Instructions: Step one foot back and bend the front knee to a 90-degree angle, keeping the back leg straight. Extend your arms parallel to the floor, palms facing down. Gaze over your front hand. Hold the pose, then switch sides.
   - Benefits: Strengthens legs, opens hips and chest, and improves stamina and balance.

Tai Chi Techniques:

1. Commencing Form:
   - Instructions: Begin with feet shoulder-width apart, arms relaxed at your sides. Slowly raise your arms to shoulder height with a gentle breath, then lower them back to your sides, focusing on smooth, flowing movements.
   - Benefits: Warms up the body, promotes relaxation, and prepares the mind for practice.

2. Grasp the Bird's Tail:
   - Instructions: From a neutral stance, step forward with one foot and extend one arm as if grasping an object. Rotate your body and shift weight as you perform this movement. Repeat on the other side.
   - Benefits: Enhances coordination, strengthens the legs, and improves the flow of Qi.

3. Single Whip:
   - Instructions: Begin with feet shoulder-width apart. Extend one arm to the side while stepping sideways with the opposite foot. Rotate your torso and shift your weight, creating a whipping motion with the arm.
   - Benefits: Improves balance, coordination, and internal energy flow.

Tips for Starting and Maintaining a Practice

1. Start Slow and Gradual:
   - Begin with basic poses or movements to build a solid foundation. Gradually increase the complexity and duration of your practice as you become more comfortable.

2. Consistency is Crucial:
   - Establish a regular practice schedule, whether it's daily or several times a week. Consistent practice helps to develop skills and integrate the benefits into your daily life.

3. Find a Qualified Instructor:
   - Consider taking classes with a certified instructor who can provide personalized guidance and feedback. This ensures correct technique and helps prevent injury.

4. Use Resources:
   - Utilize online tutorials, apps, or books to support your practice. Many resources offer detailed instructions and variations for different levels of experience.

5. Listen to Your Body:
   - Pay attention to how your body feels during practice. Modify poses or movements if you experience discomfort, and respect your limits to avoid injury.

3. Enhancing Mindfulness Through Movement

How to Integrate Yoga and Tai Chi into Daily Routines

1. Create a Dedicated Space:
   - Set up a quiet, comfortable space for practice at home. This can be a designated area with a mat or a specific room where you can focus without distractions.

2. Set a Routine:
   - Incorporate yoga or tai chi into your daily routine. Choose a time that works best for you, whether it's in the morning to start the day or in the evening to unwind.

3. Combine Practices:
   - Mix yoga and tai chi to create a varied routine. For example, you might practice yoga in the morning to stretch and energize, and tai chi in the evening for relaxation and balance.

4. Join a Community:
   - Participate in group classes or online communities to stay motivated and connect with others who share your interests. Group settings can provide support, inspiration, and additional resources.

Benefits for Mental and Physical Health

1. Mental Health:
   - Yoga and tai chi promote mental relaxation and clarity. The mindful aspect of both practices helps to reduce stress, anxiety, and depression, enhancing overall mental well-being.

2. Physical Health:
   - Regular practice improves flexibility, strength, and balance. Both yoga and tai chi support cardiovascular health, improve posture, and reduce the risk of injuries.

3. Holistic Wellness:
   - The integration of mind, body, and breath in yoga and tai chi supports a holistic approach to health. This comprehensive practice fosters a deeper connection between physical and mental wellness, leading to a more balanced and harmonious life.

By incorporating yoga and tai chi into your life, you can experience profound benefits for both body and mind. These practices offer valuable tools for enhancing mindfulness, relaxation, and overall well-being, contributing to a healthier and more balanced lifestyle.

Conclusion

Integrating Mindfulness into Daily Life

To seamlessly weave mindfulness into your daily routine, it's essential to create a personalized practice that fits your lifestyle and addresses your unique needs. Start by reflecting on what aspects of your life you want to improve through mindfulness. Are you seeking stress reduction, emotional balance, or increased focus? Identifying your goals will help you tailor your practices effectively.

Begin by selecting techniques that resonate with you. Whether you're drawn to breathing exercises, mindful eating, or yoga, choose practices that engage and benefit you. Establish a consistent schedule, starting with short, manageable sessions, and gradually increase the duration as you become more comfortable. Consistency is key to making mindfulness a natural part of your daily life.

Create a dedicated space for your mindfulness practice. This could be a quiet corner of your home where you feel comfortable and free from distractions. A serene environment enhances your ability to focus and relax during practice.

Set realistic goals to avoid feeling overwhelmed. Start with achievable objectives, such as a five-minute daily meditation, and celebrate small victories along the way. Use tools and resources like apps, online videos, or mindfulness journals to support your practice and keep you motivated.

Maintaining a mindfulness practice can be challenging due to time constraints, distractions, or lack of motivation. Address these obstacles by integrating practices into your existing routine. For instance, practice mindful breathing during breaks or mindful eating during meals. Create a routine and stick to it, and don't hesitate to seek guidance from instructors or resources if you encounter difficulties.

Long-Term Benefits and Growth

Consistent mindfulness practice yields significant long-term benefits for both mental and physical health. Over time, mindfulness helps build emotional resilience, enabling you to better manage stress and navigate life's challenges with a calm and balanced perspective. It fosters improved mental health by reducing symptoms of anxiety and depression, leading to a more positive outlook on life.

Mindfulness also enhances self-awareness, providing deeper insight into your thoughts, feelings, and behaviors. This heightened self-awareness can lead to more conscious decision-making and improved interpersonal relationships. By practicing compassion and empathy through techniques like loving-kindness meditation, you can strengthen your connections with others and improve communication.

Physically, practices such as yoga and tai chi contribute to improved flexibility, strength, and overall fitness. Regular practice supports a healthier lifestyle and helps prevent chronic conditions. The benefits extend beyond physical health, promoting a sense of overall well-being and vitality.

As you continue your mindful journey, stay curious and open to new techniques and experiences. Reflect on your progress regularly to appreciate the positive changes in your life and identify areas for further growth. Engage with mindfulness communities for support and inspiration, and be flexible in adapting your practice to fit your evolving needs.

Celebrate the milestones and progress you make in your mindfulness journey. Recognize the positive impact on your life and continue to build upon this foundation for sustained well-being. Embracing mindfulness with patience and curiosity will enrich your life and foster ongoing personal growth.

9 798335 159098